WHO SAYS?

THE FOURTH ONE

RITA MORSON

Published in 2015 by:
Stellar Books LLP
Dunham Gatehouse
Charcoal Road
Bowdon
Cheshire
WA14 4RY.

W: www.stellarbooks.co.uk
E: info@stellarbooks.co.uk
T: 0161 928 8273
Tw: @stellarbooksllp

ISBN: 978-1910275146

A copy of this book is available in the British Library.

*To Sophie, David and Simon for their
inspiration and sustaining power.
They never gave up on me.*

ACKNOWLEDGEMENTS

All my family and friends, staff at Addenbrookes and Stanmore, those who helped at the scene of the accident and those who sent me cards, good wishes and came to visit me, carrying me on my journey. Thank you especially to Michael for his key phrase of encouragement, "Who Says?"

About the Author

Rita was born in Southampton and went to school at St Benedict's Convent, Andover and West Bridgford High, Nottingham. She is married to David, has a son Simon, a granddaughter, Sophie and a sister, Barbara.

Rita worked primarily in business as a PA, but has interests in poetry, The Classics (she has an MA from the Open University) and in the fields of Christian Ecumenism and World Faiths.

Her major passion is dancing .She is now retired and maintains all of her interests and her main role of caring for and looking after Sophie.

Contents

PREFACE

On Sunday 17th July 2011, my wife Rita, our granddaughter Sophie and I were passengers in the back seat of a friend's car. It was early afternoon and we were making our way through a country route in Cambridgeshire on our way to a Garden Party. All of a sudden our friend, who was driving, swerved to miss some debris in the road and hit a van head on. My wife, who was sitting behind him, broke her neck in two places. Miraculously, in the car behind on a remote road, were two nurses, a married couple from Milton Keynes. The wife opened the boot, got inside and held Rita's head in place until the paramedic doctor arrived. The husband administered to our friend's wife in the front seat who had been hit in the eye by a broken mirror. The driver, Sophie and myself had escaped with bruising.

When I arrived at Addenbrookes Hospital in Cambridge, late on that Sunday afternoon, I was met by three surgeons who told me they must operate, as they had less than an hour to save Rita, even then there was a high likelihood that she would be paralysed from the neck down. Later that night, I was called into intensive care and miraculously the prognosis seemed hopeful as there was slight movement in her arms and legs.

I cannot thank the two nurses, the paramedic and the three surgeons highly enough for saving Rita's life.

After four days in intensive care and ten more days in an intensive care ward where the news for a recovery seemed hopeful, Rita was transferred to The Royal Orthopaedic Hospital, Stanmore, Middlesex, where after extensive tests she was told that she would never walk again. This was a devastating blow to take after the optimism at the local hospital.

This is Rita's own account of her struggle to deal with this news and to overcome it.

David Morson

PART ONE

Trauma

ADDENBROOKES

I awoke to strange noises, subdued lighting, muted voices… Muffled footsteps. What is happening? Where is David? I tried shouting but could only emit croaks. Then again oblivion, voices stronger. What has happened? Where am I? They had put me in this large, yellow capsule. I was terrified and struggled to be free - to no avail, and I cried at my helplessness.

Eventually David arrived and the explanation was a car crash. But not to worry. Everyone was OK, except for me. Sophie! Oh what of my granddaughter, Sophie! As long as Sophie was OK with no injuries whatsoever. My relief was overwhelming. The next few days were blurred for me as I sank into what must have been intensive care.

Then I left behind the shadowy figure at the end of my bed, the young man in white coat who administered to me and 'came to' in the General Ward of Addenbrookes. The nursing staff on the Ward were kind and light-hearted, and I was so happy to hear the Surgeon say,

"I don't see why you should not make a full recovery."

Oh relief as I couldn't move my body without it being painful, but the prognosis was incredibly hopeful. All I had to do was 'keep my chin up' and concentrate primarily on getting well, and going back to being Sophie's mum, as I had been since her own mother tragically died of an embolism when she was five. I believed I would be back in that role very soon. In this state of mind I was happy and also overwhelmed by the many, many words of comfort winging their way to me via David, my many visitors and Get Well cards.

My days in the hospital were peppered with viewing *"Mamma Mia"*. It was such a colourful film - beautiful scenery, catchy songs, fantastic choreography - it was my bedtime reading, and it gave a lift to my spirits. As we had individual TVs, it didn't encroach on the other patients in my ward with their viewing, so life was without any great trouble.

After nearly three weeks in hospital, a cheery young lad blithely sat beside my bed and cheerily announced he was trying to find an Orthopaedic hospital to which I could be transferred. Why do I need to transfer? I was quite happy to stay until I improved a little more. I pleaded with him why not let me stay, No, there were three other possibilities: London, Stoke Mandeville, or Sheffield. I was alarmed, all of them were so far away. A hospital on my doorstop, was surely the best option. What of visitors....? My granddaughter, and my husband? I put this to the cheery young man without effect. As it turned out, I was sent to The Royal Orthopaedic, Stanmore, Middlesex, a hospital considered the best in the country for treating patients with spinal injuries. But, of course, at that time, it was small comfort.

CARDS

The Cards, WELL, they just kept coming, nearly three hundred of them. It was a delight; it made me feel so warm; I eagerly looked forward to every evening.

How can I let people know how much they meant to me to receive them...? An idea flashed through my mind and, in my 'doodles', I came up with a bookmark. It was a way of saying a huge thank you:

> *"The cards started coming, the telephone started ringing constantly as a great wave of support, love and goodwill swept in.*
>
> *It was unbelievable, and from this came tremendous strength for me and David. Whenever I was particularly down - frightened and alone, messages on cards, visitors to my*

bedside and a deep sense of spiritual awareness came to my rescue comforted and soothed me.

I didn't need to pray, it was all done for me by those well-wishers, known and unknown.

It carried me along like riding on a great wave of energy, and almost everything I asked for was granted to me.

I cannot thank all of you enough who were part of this 'miracle', and I wanted to tell you how grateful I am and say that you were part of this amazing recovery; the wonder did not lie with me it lay in a great outpouring of love and concern that conquered all the negative elements."

But, above all, it was David's dedication to my happiness and well-being that brushed away these critical moments when I believed in the negative making it frightening and dark.

David's refusal to let me dwell on these times, coming as he did with visitors, cards and gifts made me look forward so much to his being there. However, those moments also had their amusing side. For example, when I asked him to bring in some T shirts, urging him strongly not the really good ones, whereupon he brought in my old gardening gear he found hanging in my wardrobe coupled with my well-worn but comfortable slippers.

Medical World

It was strange waking up in the morning and now part of the medical world. So very different - worlds apart. Can't walk, can't move from my position without help.

"What do you want for breakfast?"

It arrives but needs the accompanying factor of an assistant but where is she? Who would help me with eating it - seeing to others, doing other duties? Never mind, didn't feel like eating anyway.

When will I be home? But nobody said. So it was a lovely day when the surgeon who did the operation said,

"I don't see why you can't make a full recovery."

I was elated and revelled in the support of my friends. Cards kept coming and new visitors every day. My friend Tim heard of my accident and the same day travelled up from Brighton to be with me. I was so happy and basked in the concern and love emanating from the people who knew me. I didn't know, I never believed, that people liked me that much; warmth exuded from them and I felt safe. I would soon be home.

There were no visible signs of injury - all was internal so I didn't look too bad, so nothing to worry about. What is this talk of being transferred to another 'better' hospital? I was content to be in Addenbrookes, just down the road from my village, among my friends, dog 'Timmy' and always, as ever, from my granddaughter Sophie who was in my care. Sophie who lost her Mum at five years old and now saw me whisked away from the site of the accident to the hospital. And now being told I was moving yet further away. Sophie had to adjust to leaving her family, (two older sisters, an aunt and maternal grandparents) at Hemel Hempstead, to leaving her school friends and move to Henham. Gradually, so gradually, coming to terms with arrangements, and now new school, new friends. It isn't fair! They are going to send me away and there is nothing I can do about it. How is Sophie going to cope?

Everything was changing and I was deeply disconcerted. What's wrong with where I am? New department, not fully up to scratch, they said. Where will I go? Stoke Mandeville, Sheffield or London? They said they would try for London, but depends when and where a bed becomes available.

Now all the horror of the accident became apparent. I wasn't going home yet, not for some time, they said. A week or two dragged by and nothing was happening so with much trepidation I, at last, became aware that moving on meant moving away.

My time at my first hospital was over. There I had dreams, hallucinations due to the mountain of tablets I was taking and, in some strange way, I was accepting more optimistically. I would, however, miss my TV and *Mamma Mia.* This film so beautiful in its scenery and the great songs. I love dancing and the choreography was exhilarating. I vowed, one day, I will be jiving away as I've always done. Dancing was magical for me and the film lightened my day and evening. I can't remember how many times I put it on but it took me out of the world of medics, and into the world of make-believe, of beauty, and answered dreams.

Arrival at Stanmore

Told I was going to be isolated from my family. Better London than Sheffield in the wintry north or to Stoke Mandeville, home to those with more serious injuries than mine.

A day was picked to transfer me but there are no NHS ambulances available! They said,

"One has been hired so be ready soon."

The ambulance arrived in due course. Did they hire it from a film set? There it stood; a grey, grey vehicle. Two cheerful, elderly men jumped out and began assisting my departure. Surely, I thought, this is not going all the way! It looked so uncomfortable; *it was uncomfortable,* and comfort on the journey was minimal and overlooked - except for the 'cheerful Charlies'. They didn't have many words to say. It helped, though as I was able to focus on beating the pain caused mainly from the hardness of the stretcher.

Hurrah - end in sight.

However, the cheerful ones had never been to this hospital before and, leaving me forlorn in a makeshift tent, spent time in looking for Reception.

I felt so lonely. I didn't know the extent of my injury at this time, and I felt so panicky, and each mile of the journey lengthened the gap from my family and friends. I was now in an environment which I trusted would make me well again.

The cheerful Charlies eventually found 'Reception' and then their bit was done. They were going back and I was staying for how long?

Thank goodness, at last someone there to ensure my comfort. But before I could enter any part of the hospital, I had to be checked over.

"Do you feel this? Do you feel that? You will have a cup of tea soon."

A little while passed and here came a doctor and nurse to carry out tests to ensure I was clear of bugs. It was very lonesome, strangers - these people - coming and going, and now I was in another environment, another set of people. Where was I now? I don't know this part of the world. All I knew was that EVERYTHING was different and my sense of loss was heightened by this fact.

Although my encounter with the ambulance people was slight, they knew the same familiar places as I did and this connection brought some degree of comfort. Now I was on my own again.

What Do You Want?

My first experience of non-care by staff was at my first night-time. Lights out, everything quiet, still paralysed from accident. Oh what does that mean? Am I going to be like this for always? Was the message from my local hospital that there was no reason why I could not make a full recovery really true?

I'm getting cold and colder. Oh for a brief, comforting hand on my forehead... (*How is Sophie doing?*) Oh for assurance from a friendly, concerned, albeit stranger. Next best thing picturing Sophie and David missing me but safe at home with Timmy the dog. Getting uncomfortable again as blankets have a will of their own. Can't sleep, blankets still not responding to my weak efforts to control them. Comfort!! Night bell, of course! Nurses had assured me, prior to 'lights out' that an emergency bell was there for a night nurse should I be uncomfortable or for any reason or need. Unable to get warm, blankets not responding still. In fact I was pushing them away! Oh, a night nurse, YES, they would probably tell me off for getting in a pickle and not letting them know.

Heigh-ho, bell pushed, no reply, probably in loo or something, another push of bell, footsteps coming, a nurse approaching a bit hurriedly. Curtains flung back, an angry voice spits out,

"WHAT DO YOU WANT?"

Surprise made me silent momentarily then:

"How dare you speak to me like that!" came tumbling out of my mouth. Were they cross because I had interrupted their TV programme? But I was a 'new' patient still in shock.

How could our "angels" behave like that? It seemed as though they were drawing up battle lines and had to deal with me - let me know that they are in charge - bells are there not to be rung - was I going to be one of the awkward patients?

FIRST FEW DAYS AT STANMORE

Everyone seemed to be busy, except me. I lay there wondering what to do. I watched nurses come and nurses go but no-one stopped to help. A bath had been promised on a new piece of equipment. In came trolley propelled by nursing assistant and away went assistant, leaving trolley to me. Being new I didn't know if there were rules to be followed, all I know is that thirty minutes later it was still trolley and me. So I lay like waiting for the chop. Thing is I can't do anything for myself. Towels were draped over me for dignity more than for warmth so we waited, trolley and me, for reappearance of our nurse.

A little Filipino lady with a bright, broad smile came to administer to my needs and to help my dressing and change my bed linen. Her lovely smile, the warmth that emanated from her gave me confidence and reassurance. However, without warning, pillow whipped from under my neck. I was startled and horrified as my main injury was the two broken bones in my neck. Explained this to my Filipino friend.

Hurrah: she now understands....still smiling... nodding her head.

Next day: Oh no! Pillow whipped away more forcefully than before. Again: I clutched pillow to me but lost my grip. To her alarm, I demanded to see the Ward Sister. Guilt flooded through me.

It wasn't "smilie's" fault. She didn't know what the matter was. She didn't speak English!

The Ward Sister tried to be conciliatory and later called a Staff Meeting to enquire whether I would be prepared to give her another chance. But I couldn't do that and this time, I held my ground. However, the dear little lady whenever we met again after this would give me a beautiful smile, no rancour in her at all.

In all this I must have been suffering from shock with regard to change in my circumstances. *Is Sophie all right?* I had been promised a bath. Instead I was still waiting. I know I will attract the attention of a nurse. Eventually I did this only to be told they were too busy - too busy even to be friendly? I tried to understand. Eventually we all joined up, nurse assistant, trolley and me, and thus was the beginning of my stay at The Royal

Orthopaedic Hospital and yearning every day to be with my family and friends.

We awoke to breakfast in the early hours of the day and thereon it was a continuous subdued bustle that one associated with hospital ward atmosphere as one sees on TV or cinema and disappointed that "cosseting" was not on the cards anymore. We had to queue for bathing, after which came physio (if you were lucky) as quite often schedules were encroached upon. I used to get so upset when this occurred as it affected my "going home" date.

Rest Room

A Newcomer - hurrah - now we can have some fresh information. Must ask her all about her injuries - how was her operation? Their faces lit up. What sort of injuries did you sustain?

"Well, it does get better dear," was said to my fear of never walking again. They wanted to know the extent of my injuries. Why didn't I? I had to wheel away. I couldn't accept their foregone conclusions and seemingly looking ahead to a life of immobility.

Well both the Consultant and Doctor had explained it fully,

"I cannot say you will make any further improvement," and the Doctor said,

"There are benefits, you know. You can still go abroad on holidays as there are travel agents who cater especially for the disabled."

Well there you are!

Nearing meal times you will find us dutifully lining up patiently awaiting our pre-ordered meal. The Rest Room was turned now into a canteen. A lump in my throat and a tear in my eye, I entered into the 'medical world.' The so-called Rest Room was a nightmare for me. They wanted to be friendly and helpful, I was wanting instead an optimistic view. But with a knowing look and a sympathetic smile, they labelled me "in denial".

NO! I do not want to talk about my accident.

NO! I do not want any travel agent to assist me to arrange a holiday for the disabled.

YES! I would like a respectful acknowledgment of my need to be silent.

YES! I would like an understanding of wanting to be alone.

THE POOL

"Would you like a dip in the Pool today?" said the Doctor, to which I replied that however enticing, I did not have enough support to do that.

"Oh yes, we now have a beautiful, modern pool in which wheel chairs have been adapted to go under water."

Sounds good, give it a try. It felt strange being able to use parts of my body otherwise paralysed. I will just check with the Doctor that my neck injury would not be damaged by such exercise.

It was decided that on the side of caution perhaps I ought to curtail this exercise. I was then deposited at the side of the pool in my wet bathing costume awaiting an attendant to dry me and take me back to my warm, comfortable bed. The time dragged on! In my weakened state I was anxious that I might catch some bug or other. Reminded Nursing Staff I was still around and needed drying and looking after........ Waiting .... felt again a sense of acute loneliness in that I had to 'keep an eye on things' myself................

Waited......................

Now <u>two hours</u> gone by.

At long last an attendant. It was explained that this long wait was due to the fact that the pool was shared with the general public and thus they had first call on its facilities. It seemed ludicrous to me that people in delicate health should be allowed to suffer, not only from the mental discomfort of being undressed by the side of the pool, but the added risk of "catching something".

The only comfort was the cries of delight from the children as they splashed about enjoying their games. So, my five minute "dip" led to a time of "two hours" reflection, leading to feelings of aloneness and insecurity. So much for my treat in the pool.

By now I was getting colder. Reminded nurses I was still around! In my misery, no-one seemed to be looking after my needs and all I can do is wait. Finally, I was washed and then taken back to my ward.

THE FOURTH ONE

He couldn't look me in the eye, that composed consultant.

"We have done all the tests..." and then a brief summary of results. I looked eagerly at him. I was not ready to hear his cold comments. I was waiting for his words of hope. He turned his head away, nonchalantly sucking on the end of his pencil and deliberately avoiding my gaze, and then told me,

"WE ARE AFRAID YOU WILL NOT WALK AGAIN."

I looked at him in disbelief.

That day began with me being quite excited. I had some control of my legs, everyone was so cheerful.

"Rita, you are remarkable, you are recovering so well," and other words of comfort. I would perhaps now be told when that wonderful day of discharge would come around.

A little apprehensive but David was there too and the sun was shining. The consultant mechanically spoke now in medical terms. I could even be home for Christmas. I would be in hospital for possibly four months, five months away. The length of stay was not only due to treatment of other injuries but mainly to teach me how to live my life in a wheelchair in the world of the disabled. Rita, of the strongly independent nature, had now to look to others to help her live.

"We will teach you in our Rehab Unit."

But what of Sophie? I couldn't be her Mum anymore. Can't bear to give her up. We had such a good relationship then. I will **not** give her up. I asked the Consultant if there was anyone who had my injuries and recovered. He replied - in all his years, only three had left the Rehab Unit walking. I gritted my teeth,

"I WILL BE THE Fourth."

Interview over, David wheeled me away into the sunlit corridor and then my resolve went and I sobbed. David buried his head in his hands and through his tears said,

"Oh Sweetheart, we will face this together."

"WHO SAYS?"

Michael, a good, old practical friend, who was many times to accompany David on his journey to and from the hospital and thereby lifting the burden of driving. David who was unfailing in his care and Michael who quashed any adverse thinking and was a true inspiration.

"Sorry, Michael, feel out of sorts today."

"Oh dear, why?"

"I'm not going to walk again."

"Who says?"

"Consultant and doctor."

"**Who says**?"

"They have the results from examination, the experts say I won't walk again."

"Who says?"

I looked closely at him. He had a bland expression ...confidence oozing from him.

"**Who says?**"

"YES, Michael WHO SAYS?"

Michael and me to start with says it! I WILL get better! I WILL WALK AGAIN!

Michael reminded me of the power of prayer from which the 300 plus cards had generated a warmth of feeling which had carried me forward on a wave of energy. All the visitors building a wall of love around me; concern and prayers, prayers, prayers for me from those in New York, Belgium, USA, Ireland, Australia, Ghana….. I **need** to walk again for love of Sophie. I'm her Mum since her own Mum died a few years ago. I can't let her down. I will walk again!!

I recall my time at Addenbrookes and the surgeon who operated on me there and remembered his words to me: "*I can't see why you won't make a full recovery.*"

But it was the Consultant here, the Consultant who carried out the tests - it was he who had the evidence to support his findings.

DOLDRUMS DAY

Nothing is right today. Feeling despondent, feeling sad at the changes in my circumstances; can't read, can't walk, most of all can't dance, just feeling as if I have changed worlds. Bright and breezy carer comes bustling in:

"Now, I think, Rita, you would like to do some gardening?"

No thanks, not today, want to be on my own. (Angry that they don't understand.) Can I share my anger? No!

Everyone is busy pushing their little trowels into little squares of earth made accessible by raising the level of the table.

"No, I don't want to do any bloody gardening and I am not going to spend my remaining years as a spectator on life!"

They nod wisely to each other: "in denial".

The doctor in charge of me came to see how I was getting on and airily remarked what good disabled holidays there are now for such as me.

I shall never forget the gardening scene - so depressing - and my horrified thoughts that this was it and my gardening was going to be my sole outlet. These people looked happy on it, but it was not for me. I threw down my trowel and asked to be taken back to my ward. They never asked me again!

NIGHT VISITORS

Mini miracles when my 'angels' knew my strength was weakening and were there for me in the form of visitors: feeling down nearing time for 'lights out', deeply aware of disabilities.

Feeling cold - drab surroundings, can't lift myself out of it BUT who is this tapping at the window during out of hours? And there is Semira, my Ba'hai friend, miles from home, thought she would pop-in.

Now I'm laughing, now I'm giggling - thank you Semira.

Panicky with results showing certain areas not functioning and medical staff ready to perform operation BUT who is that on the line? Anthea, my Quaker friend offering words of comfort, and away goes the fear and the problem!

Now I'm laughing and at ease.

Mentally finding it difficult to sustain a bright smile. Feeling inadequate, a burden to others, BUT who is this coming into the Ward with a positive attitude, makes my heart respond?

Now I'm chuckling, and I'm feeling mentally strong.

It's Amanda - all the way from Cambridge.

Tonight, dreading the dark, frightening is the future BUT who is this sweeping into the 'closed' area of reception? It's Sister Judith!

"Just thought I would pop-in to see how you are, dear."

The force of her amazing personality sweeping away any opposition she may have met. Sister Judith a sparkling, loveable nun in a wheel-chair. She exuded love and aliveness. She couldn't be suppressed which doesn't mean she couldn't see pain. She was tender but firm. She left me with a sense of achievement to build on.

Now I'm smiling.

Now I'm wanting to fight with a smile in my heart BUT who is this 'night visitor' peeping around the ward? It looks like Pam! It can't be Pam, she doesn't visit; she can't as she gets too nervous away from home. **IT IS PAM....!** Who has travelled from Hemel Hempstead which must have cost her many a pang.

Now I'm elated.

A visit from Pam is special as it costs so much more. I am grateful for all my lovely friends. Those individuals mentioned above reflect all areas who came to my bedside.

However, words cannot be said enough regarding the dedication from David, my husband. Every evening he was there to comfort and help me cope, to reassure me, to make sure I lacked nothing in the material as well as the mental sense. I was anxious that he was coming every day as it was a three hour journey and there was Sophie to consider. Could he sustain it? He could…with the help of McDonalds'…. Without his cheerfulness, I could not have managed!

MENUS

"What would you like tomorrow for lunch/dinner?"

For ease of administration one had to order one's food the day before. No big deal; I'll remember this. The meals were OK, not exciting but adequate. After a week or two I noticed two menus were available and enquired if I could choose a meal from the more exotic one being served.

"Could I have one of those tomorrow?"

"Of course."

So next day I tucked into my curry which, after the blandness of European food, was absolutely delicious. So ordered another curry for the next meal.

"Are you sure I ordered curry again? Did I order curry for lunch? Perhaps it was dinner?"

The trouble is that with ordering 24 hours in advance one didn't always remember what order they came in. Did I order the day following lunch then or perhaps it was dinner? At the time I believed I wouldn't forget, so next meal time.....

"Are you *sure* I made that choice? Curry again?"

"Oh yes, paper to prove it."

So I dig into another curry!

It was visiting time so David came along and we visited the little secluded part of the hospital garden. Tummy rumbled. Oh dear, better make for the loo quickly. Oh dear, too late....

"David, can you fetch some paper!"

"David, where can I go....?" Then:

"Quickly, David - loads of paper! Find some more!"

It's coming out of my shoes!!!

How can I have generated so much?

We now had tons of soiled paper which I was desperate to dispose of.

Hark, is someone coming? They would see me with diarrhoea spilling over into my shoes, and a huge amount of soiled paper by me. No, I was OK. No-one coming but what do I do? I didn't want to reveal myself for all the world to see. My eyes fell on a garden waste bag, half full and eagerly I filled it up with David looking on quite dazed. I can't imagine what the gardener must have thought - pretty strong manure they are making today, but I was saved from the awful ordeal, and dear David was doing his very best to clean away all traces of diarrhoea and leaving me with some sort of dignity.

C'MON

Today, however, feeling depressed by it all: overlooked, a nuisance, discomfort, despairing. I remember looking up at the stormy sky and wondering what it was all about; the suddenness of my mishap and where would it end. I was bewildered, frightened as well.

I wasn't used to people doing things for me or leading me along. I have often thought that some time in hospital, being waited upon and cosseted, was to be envied without, of course, the discomforts of pain and imagined a world as in the days depicted by Hattie Jacques, where patients were the main thought and were there to comfort and be their 'angel'.

But what is coming now? A changeover of nursing personnel? Down the ward swings my particular 'angels' with whom I felt safe under their collective care.

Trevor from Roumania, smiling, relaxed.

"I am here to look after you."

Maria also from Roumania, did mainly night shift, and whose first task was always cups of tea for everyone around. It was Maria with whom I shared my concerns regarding Sophie and I learnt of her hopes and fears for her little twin girls.

Cecile! Oh Cecile originally from Senegal, a very special angel who understood my mental as well as my physical needs. What can I say about this particular person? She was the nurse of my dreams - the Hattie Jacques of the ward. Nothing too much trouble; concerned if I was uncomfortable. She knew I was troubled about having to administer to myself and found it difficult to learn. She cosseted and cared for me - coming in before she needed to and gentle with helping me insert the necessary tubes. Cecile, who will always remain in my memory as an angel. Why? Her utter kindness helped my recovery. I will always remember how she kept to her promises. ("I'll be here tomorrow half an hour early to help you along.") Doing the administering for me at times, to take over when I just couldn't manage. Helped me more than she should. Other nurses suspicious, and believed that by helping me so well made their jobs busier than they liked.

Trevor, who happened to be in the ward when one of the physio's was passing through and took to heart their remark that I should be encouraged to move from bed to chair.

"C'mon…" Trevor said….. Wretched man. He's too insistent…

"I don't feel well Trevor…"

"C'mon…"

"I'll do it tomorrow… Promise I'll do it in the morning…"

"C'mon….."

"Oh very well…." I broke under his stronger will.

But….Thank you….Thank you Trevor. I sank back in to my bed and chair. I did it! With Trevor's persistence, **my first steps**! Trevor knew I could do it and it was another arrow in my bow that I proudly told everyone of course!

So, angels do abound, sometimes difficult to find, but thanks and love to those who see it as their vocation, to administer and negate the pain, not only physical but mental and bring cheer to bewildered, frightened people, like myself.

THE MARVELLOUS BAND OF PHYSIOS

Everyone a delight. So dedicated to those sent to them for healing. They surely need successes as a great many will never walk or regain their mobility, and the sadness that surrounds these people must, at times, be unbearable to witness. Their hopes and their dreams will have been shattered and they have to build again, to have other dreams. It must be like one hears of funeral parlours, they are the joliest places in which to work, and, certainly the Physio Department was in that category as goodwill abounded.

Natasha, Chief Physio said,

"I have booked a photographer for you tomorrow morning to film where you are going wrong in trying to walk again."

"OK, will be here and try not to be late."

(Missed appointments mainly due to ablutions carried out by staff.) Many a time I was deeply upset for I knew that every successful effort, everything new asked of me, the patient was a step nearer to going home. For me this meant my husband, my granddaughter and Timmy, our dog.

I duly arrived next morning in the gymnasium. They were setting up the props, the bars which I was to walk between.

"Right now, Rita, do your best...."

I concentrated all my energy, thinking strongly for Sophie. Then slowly but surely my efforts for the sake of Sophie came to an end with Natasha open-mouthed looking at me.

"Rita how can you do this to me? I've engaged a photographer to help you and you have just walked <u>*perfectly*</u>*!"*

<u>*The miracle had happened!!! I will be the fourth one to walk out of here.*</u>

<u>*Thank you Natasha!!!...*</u>

<u>*Thank you all!!!*</u>

Eager to show my prowess, I asked two nurses to accompany me out of my ward using just my two sticks. Slowly, painfully I edged my way out and was determined to get as far as the Reception Desk, only a little distance away.

There was a shout. People turned around. The nurses and staff on the Reception Desk were clapping and... I fell flat on my face!

LEAVING

I want to go home! They said all being well, I could leave before Christmas….. Months away yet and I want to go now! I was finding it difficult "keeping up appearances" and missed my family and friends acutely.

"Do you think it could be considered? I really will be good - like taking loads of rest…" (That was no problem with David around.)

There were others in the ward who dreaded going home frightened, I believe, because of lack of balance and sustaining further injury. But, I asked for a meeting of all my carers and told them, I would like to be home for Sophie's half term in October. To my surprise they agreed…. no problem!

I was on my way!

PART TWO

Turning Around

Turning/Turnaround

To recall, it was a Sunday afternoon in July and we were merrily bowling along in the car through quiet country lanes to Virginia's garden party. An annual event to raise money for an orphanage. We eagerly looked forward to meeting up again with old friends and perhaps finding new ones. The setting in Virginia's glorious gardens made the prospect of it being a most delightful afternoon.

This particular year we accepted a lift from friends also from the same village. The day was bright, tranquil, the fields and birds singing and flowers blooming..... CRASH..... To avoid debris in the road, the driver had swerved into the path of a van.... Silence.... Then voices muffled. I asked someone to help me as I could not move my head. More voices, then a dusty pink atmosphere came into my consciousness, and I felt myself drifting away into total darkness........

Another year on now before I pick up my pen to continue my thoughts from my hospital bed. What is the message I have? Why do I have a need to write of it? What is new? Have I lost something precious in the intervening year? Have I found my 'angel', my friends again, my inspirational reflections?

I would like to reach out to those who lack hope and to find with you a beautiful way of living. To life....

- I would like to give a resounding YES!
- to love my life in spite of mishaps.................
- to don't take 'no' for an answer without exploring further
- to share with others our hopes, our dreams, our <u>trust</u>
- to recognise the false acceptance of facts - the message I have is *HOPE.*

MY GUARDIAN ANGEL

She came to me in the night, she was there in the murmuring voices, in the lights, in the hurried gestures *but wait* she was there at the scene of the accident! I saw a distressed Sophie, puzzled but unhurt, checking on the other passengers. I heard normal voices - myself asking for help as I couldn't lift my head. Then total blackness and silence. Gone was the dusty-pink atmosphere and myself viewing the scene from a distance like a "faraway" vista from on high.

Noises, something happening, where was I? Where is David? - Strangers - were, trying to get me into a yellow machine which clonked threateningly. No! No! No! Leave me be but I could not fight against them anymore, so I gave way to my struggling and cried at the terror I was feeling. Can't make it out - someone was talking to me - telling me that I would survive.

But it may mean I would be paralysed from the neck down. No, I couldn't agree to that. I do not want to face the future. Let me be. I choose to go – I was drifting around a bend and there was no fear in me.

Then a rapid change of scene - myself seeing myself on a trolley being pushed along in a great rush. Strange that I was in two places at once. You looked up at me and told me I would make a full recovery and I said that on that promise I would not go away.

You were a plump little lady with dark hair and an earnest expression.

In the moments after my 'return' I couldn't piece together the scenario and it wasn't until many weeks later after that I realised that I had momentary died and I was two personalities for that time of body and spirit. It later proved as in my psychological report that such an incident was plausible. (It was also then that I recognised my Guardian Angel who promised she would be with me always. She sits at the turn of a staircase and thoughts come in to my mind and answers are given to my queries put to her.)

Returning/Turn About

Returning, mentally, to the scene of the accident, it was one I knew little about - the horror of it was within me until full consciousness came a while later. Even so, I did not wish to talk about it then. (It only came after I returned home some four months later.)

However, some curiosity made me ask if paper cuttings, such as local press, could be kept in case I felt a need to understand my 'miraculous' recovery. I learnt then how indebted I was, for my life, to a series of very concerned people who knew how to react in a crisis and, of course, my angels who were always with me: the two paramedics who were travelling to a venue for a day out with family and knew that any movement by me or anyone else was critical to my survival.

One of the paramedics crawled into the back of the car and for over an hour held my head securely, while the Fire Brigade, cut off the roof of the car to release me, and another fireman who gave a teddy bear to Sophie to soften the seriousness of the situation for her. The helicopter hovering overhead in case it was needed and wrapping me up like a 'mummy' to avoid any adverse movement.

All this happened on a bright sunny afternoon on a Sunday; the three people in the following car who looked after Sophie while everybody was looking after me. The ambulance personnel who raced to our local hospital as an operation was crucial to my survival.

All these people with their concerns helped me eventually to turn around and find my Guardian Angel. In turning around, I see various people (angels) who were close to me, comforting me in my confused state.

I arrived at the hospital where my husband was told an operation was essential and three surgeons were dressed awaiting his consent to operate. David was advised that there was a possibility that I may be paralysed from the neck down. "Hearing" such conditions, I did not want to survive. My Guardian Angel then assured me I wouldn't have to,

"You will make a full recovery."

My shining ones were there - Angels, Angels everywhere.

MUSINGS

When lying on my hospital bed and musing on the tremendous changes in my life and how I felt supported by friends, I was deeply grateful. There was a chance, a real chance that things could turn around for me and the book mark in thanks for that support was a powerful way of me reaching out to many people.

They never thought I would walk again. Their decision was final, so my many pleas to be treated differently fell on deaf ears. Amanda, my friend from Cambridge, went from pillar to post searching for me because she was told that I would not be in that Ward, that's for those who can walk. I was given forms to fill in. Why? I could apply for numerous things such as a stair lift, bath appliances, also I could go on a training course. I protested (except for Blue Badge!)

Going Home

The day eventually dawned when it was "going home" time. **Elated! Out of hospital. On to real home.**

It brought home to me the importance of how we are all needful of our "family" whether biological or not, it covers those who are our special friends.

Lovely, David and Michael came to reclaim me, taking me first to *McDonalds*, then to real home. So strange the walking in public. In hospital everyone had some form of helpful apparatus but this time, I was still in the medical world of the disabled and just thanking my angels and friends for my continued success. All of this, however, meant an increase in David's responsibility to myself and Sophie. David was eager to help in every way but we both knew that our capacities were limited. The lighter side that David and I experienced and many a merry moment when we looked at how he tried to help me dress, and goodness knows how he managed to get all the clothes back to front, inside out, and goodness knows, only a grateful and untruthful wife could call concoctions, great. But these happenings brought David and myself closer. There was Sophie oblivious to the variety of colour in her gear, and very happy to be taken to McDonalds most days of the week - it helped David to cope to have this fall-back.

Home is getting nearer, familiar sights passed and then there was my home in Henham, bedecked with banner WELCOME HOME on doorway and bottles of wine. And then Timmy, our dog, heard my voice and came like a bullet out of a gun, completely berserk so that people had to prise him away from me.

The Voice of Henham

The voice of Henham sounded in its great acts of kindness when people left innumerable Shepherds Pies to help David along. Words of welcome from the pulpit when our local Vicar, on behalf of his parishioners, made the three hour trip to see how I was getting on.

"Well, what brings you to this area?" I cheerily asked.

"To see you, of course," was the reply, "so that I can give first hand news of your progress."

Another voice which sent good wishes in a card:

"You don't know me but you are from our village..."

My first Sunday, Father Joe, our priest, who led the congregation in clapping me "home".

Further recollections that kept me wondering: new attitudes within myself of quietude, reflection, made me happy. A precious gift.

Leaving the world in full summer and wondering why I needed winter clothing, made me confused. Never wanted to see press cuttings or talk about accident. Made me feel insecure.

During my hospital time cried three times; firstly under pressure to enter a 'drum' which terrified me, then the indignity of daily washing made me sob bitterly and then despair at being told,

"You will never walk again."

I was to remember the words of encouragement, "Who says?" from our dear friend Michael who dared to question and allowed me to explore the possibilities of returning to full health.

One year later I recall with much wonder what was said to me by the surgeon from Addenbrookes after my operation, when he took my hand and said, "You have made my day!" in seeing my efforts to walk and that maybe, maybe I can make a full recovery. He said that he only had less than an hour to save me and that my life had been in the balance.

The doctor attending the consultant could not believe her eyes and collapsed back on to her chair repeating, "I'm so happy, I'm so happy!"

And I had the biggest of smiles on my face in sheer delight at their reception.

I had promised to keep up exercises: that is ballet!

I have always had a passion for ballet and had attended weekly lessons at the local school of Dance before the accident.

"Oh no," they said "that would not be possible."

"Pardon me!.... Ahem…."

Tut Tut! Who is that with ballet shoes swinging away to classical music, bumping along at the back of the room….? ME!

My relationship with Sophie changed slowly but surely as in reply to a query,

"Are you looking after your Nana?" replied,

"No, she should be looking after me!"

"Quite right."

The Gas Man Cometh!

Early one morning the gas man came to call. I explained to him that I found it difficult to walk due to a car crash which had left me with two broken bones in my neck among other injuries and that was the reason I took so long to answer the door. He said that he was a part-time fireman and remembered the crash well on hearing the location.

The crash was now over a year ago, but the gas man talked as if it were yesterday. I was the talk of the fire station. Why?

He remembered that I had been classed as a "goner". But here I am alive, looking relaxed, looking ahead. He was full of admiration.

But curiously "miraculous" was a title that most people were using about my recovery: various medical staff at the hospital, those at the local surgery, friends near and far.

All were delighted to see a "transformed" Rita. Prayers were indeed working.

Up until the meeting with the gas man/ fireman, I had found it difficult to talk about the actual incident and shied away from the publicity this engendered.

I now can. With the appearance on the scene of the fireman, have learnt to look at it with wondering eyes, but "time being a great healer" and growing acceptance.

Conclusions

What are my feelings telling me now? I trust I am slowly moving towards a deeper spiritual happening. My hope is that I will be able to make this journey alongside others and explore our future days. These present days are days of renewal and gradually I am returning to full recovery - as promised.

Future days are days of learning to love my life instead of being apprehensive about what the day will bring and to help Sophie fulfill her future potential.

When I asked in prayer for greater understanding, thoughts came winging to me of quietude, reflection, meditation but, most of all, of being happy.

Every now and then I would experience a beautiful feeling; one of joy, one of wonder and puzzlement as to where it was leading me. I am still in that puzzle, but cherish the mystery and the gentleness.

WHO SAYS?